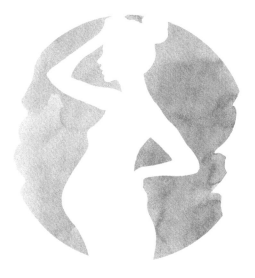

A PRACTICAL GUIDE ON GESTATIONAL DIABETES

Ten things you need to know

Pinner Green Books
Copyright @ 2018 Pinner Green
Books. All rights reserved.

Follow us on Instagram:
about_gestational_diabetes

INTRODUCTION

Being diagnosed with gestational diabetes can be shocking and upsetting. It can also be bewildering – there's a lot to learn and you can feel lost in all the information. Where do you start? This book is a good place!

I wrote this guide to help women get to grips with what they need to know - quickly. When I was diagnosed back in 2020, I found that even though there was a lot of information available it was outdated.

I found hospital brochures and some websites saying for example, low fat or fat free yoghurts were good to eat! Contradicting what many online wellness gurus have been saying for the past few years: natural full fat yoghurt is better for you. It has more nutrients, more probiotics, less additives and sweeteners and will keep you feeling fuller.

Confusing and unhelpful to say the least!

It took me a while to get the hang of it - when to test, what to eat, how to adjust meals, how much exercise I needed. I'm going to share with you everything I learnt along the way. This book isn't going to focus on the science, risks or statistics.

This book is more of a practical guide to help you navigate through this quickly and help you on your path to having a healthy pregnancy and baby.

One important note before we dive in: the information here is shared for educational purposes and does not replace the advice from your Medical Practitioner. Every individual is unique and what works for one person may not work for another. Your health should always be managed in consultation with a Healthcare Professional who can provide personalised guidance and support.

CONTENTS

CHAPTER 1

IT'S NOT YOUR FAULT

You have gestational diabetes. Now what?

It's normal to feel shaken, upset and guilty when you first get diagnosed with gestational diabetes.

Pregnancy is complicated enough, your body is going through so many changes, it's busy making a human, hormones are chaotic, you are adjusting to your new body, there are new emotions and you are preparing to be a parent. Alongside this, there's appointments, baby gear to buy, maternity leave to sort. It's a minefield, lots of new things happening all at once. It is already A LOT and now there's something new to learn about and deal with - gestational diabetes.

Unhelpful thoughts like: is it something I did? could I have prevented this from happening? am I going to hurt my baby may also be creeping into your mind.

But you know what, it's not your fault and it's important to know that and move forward.

- You don't get gestational diabetes because you ate too much sugar.
- People who have a normal BMI, are not overweight can also suffer from gestational diabetes.
- No one really understands why it happens.

Pregnancy does not last long, by the time you've been diagnosed you'll probably only have about 12-16 weeks left until you meet your new little baby. You need to become knowledgeable quickly, and gain some control back.

TIPS

- Be kind to yourself.
- To help alleviate feelings of shock and guilt try talking to friends/family, give meditation or affirmations a go, or seek professional counselling.

CHAPTER 2

GESTATIONAL DIABETES

There is lots of information online about what gestational diabetes is. The purpose here is to give you a basic overview of what is happening and not a deep dive science lesson.

Gestational diabetes occurs during pregnancy when the body becomes insulin resistance. Insulin is a hormone produced by the pancreas and it helps your body use sugar (glucose from carbohydrates) for energy.

In gestational diabetes a hormone made by your placenta prevents your body from using insulin correctly. Because insulin is not working as effectively as normal it leads to high blood sugar.

No one knows why this happens but there are associated risk factors such as:
- High blood pressure
- Family history of diabetes
- Excess body weight, especially if concentrated around the abdomen

- Ethnicity, including African-American, Hispanic, Native American, Asian-American, South Asian, Middle Eastern
- Women with polycystic ovary syndrome or prediabetes

High blood sugar is not good for you or your baby. There is risk of possible complications but with careful management they are usually preventable. Things your Healthcare team will make you aware of (and monitor) include the baby:

- being larger than usual
- arriving earlier than planned
- having low blood sugar when born

You may be affected in the following ways:

- high blood pressure
- more likely to develop type 2 diabetes later in life

It's important to know that most women with gestational diabetes will have a healthy pregnancy and baby. Gestational diabetes will usually disappear shortly after birth.

CHAPTER 3

GLUCOSE MONITOR READINGS

You will be asked to monitor your blood sugar levels on a regular basis and to keep a diary. You will most likely get an electronic blood glucose meter, where you will have to prick your finger and place a small amount of blood onto a test strip which will then be placed into the meter. After a few seconds you will get a reading.

Your Healthcare Practitioner will advise on what your blood sugar levels should be but generally:

	Most common unit used in: UK, Australia, UK, Canada	Most common unit used in: US, France, India
Fasting levels	<5.3 mmol/l	95 mg/dL
One hour after meal	<7.8 mmol/l	<140 mg/dL
Two hours after meal	<6.7 mmol/l	<120 mg/dL

Your Healthcare Practitioner will tell you when to take your readings but below are the most common times to test your blood sugar levels.

1. When you wake up and before you eat anything (this is a fasting reading)

When you don't eat for a long period of time like overnight, your liver releases glucose for energy. When you have gestational diabetes, this can mean your fasting glucose reading can be higher than it should be in the mornings and that's why it is important to monitor.

If you find your fasting reading is higher than 5.3 mmol/l or 95mg/dL try making some adjustments such as:

- Have a snack before bedtime (e.g. cheese with oatcakes, nuts with natural Greek yoghurt, apple/pear with cheese)
- Reduce the fasting time overnight
- Avoid carb heavy meals in the evening
- Analyse your diet and see if you are getting enough of the good carbs? Too little carbohydrates may also cause an increase.
- Try and get a good night's sleep
- Make sure you are hydrated
- Check your stress levels (read the section titled stress reduction)

2. Right before a meal (also called pre-prandial)

In some instances, your Healthcare Practitioner may also advise you to take readings before the meal. This is useful, particularly at the beginning of your journey as it will help give you a better picture of how the food is impacting your blood sugar levels.

3. 1 or 2 hours after your meal (also called postprandial)
This will show the level of sugar in your blood after you've eaten and indicate how your body responded to that meal. It reveals how well (or not so well) your body processed the carbohydrates and uses insulin. The aim is to keep this below 7.8 mmol/l or 140 mg/dL.

TIPS

- You'll be taking several readings every day and your fingers can get quite sore with all the pricking. Remember to alternate fingers and the location each time.
- You may find certain fingers are better at drawing blood than others. I found the plushest part of my ring finger the best and my little finger the worst!
- Make sure your hands are warm. It will improve blood circulation.
- Thoroughly wash your hands using soap and warm water and use a clean towel to dry your hands on. Any residue on your hands can give incorrect results.
- Keep your testing kit, diary and pen in a convenient location. Going up and down the stairs can get quite challenging over the course of a pregnancy. I found a suitable spot in my kitchen and kept everything there.

CHAPTER 4

ADJUSTMENTS TO DIET

Ok, let's get down to the nitty gritty – what to eat. There are two straightforward rules to follow.

One: eat real, unprocessed (or minimally processed) food. General rule of thumb: if it was made in a factory, don't eat it (or limit it) and stick to natures food.

There are exceptions of course, so get good at reading food labels. Try and avoid if:

- there are more than five ingredients and contains lots of preservatives, flavourings.
- you don't recognise the ingredients; there are things listed on the label that you wouldn't use if you were cooking at home.
- if sugar is one of the first 3 ingredients mentioned in the list. This includes glucose, syrup, artificial sweeteners, corn syrup.
- it's made with unhealthy oils such as soybean, corn, canola, rapeseed, sunflower and safflower.

Examples of foods that are usually minimally processed and beneficial to include in your diet are things like:

- Natural full fat Greek yoghurt
- Dairy milk
- Cheese
- Cottage cheese
- Frozen fruit and vegetables
- Some types of sourdough (but check ingredients using the guidelines above)
- Tofu / tempeh
- Cold pressed oils, grass fed butter

But please check the labels as regulations vary from country to country.

Carbohydrates get a lot of bad press, and yes, the usual suspects like pasta, white bread, cakes, biscuits (anything made with white refined flour) can cause high blood sugar and are best avoided (or drastically reduced and paired with fat/protein). However, good carbohydrates are still important to include in your diet. You should incorporate carbohydrates like:

- Quinoa
- Buckwheat
- Beans
- Lentils
- Chickpeas

Two: how you plate your food

This is an easy way to make sure you are having a balance diet and getting the nutrients you and your baby need. This strategy actually makes meal planning easier especially for families as you can still have the same meal just plate it as shown below.

Basically, vegetable should make up half your plate, protein a quarter and fats and carbs one eighth each.

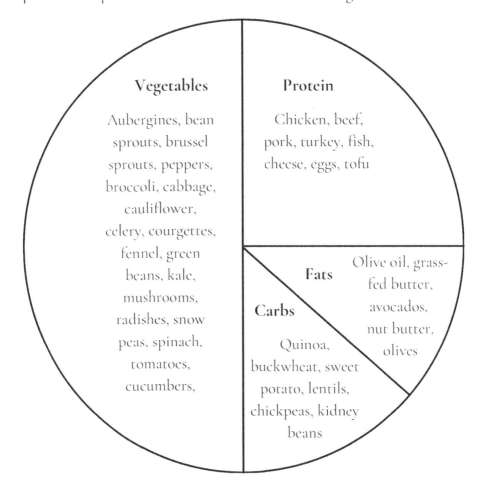

Vegetables

Aubergines, bean sprouts, brussel sprouts, peppers, broccoli, cabbage, cauliflower, celery, courgettes, fennel, green beans, kale, mushrooms, radishes, snow peas, spinach, tomatoes, cucumbers,

Protein

Chicken, beef, pork, turkey, fish, cheese, eggs, tofu

Fats

Olive oil, grass-fed butter, avocados, nut butter, olives

Carbs

Quinoa, buckwheat, sweet potato, lentils, chickpeas, kidney beans

- The order in which you eat your food impacts your blood sugar levels. The best order in which to eat your meal is vegetables first, then protein and carbohydrates last. This order will result in a smaller increase in blood sugar levels.
- Mix a tablespoon of apple cider vinegar in a glass of water and drink before your meal. Research shows that it reduces blood sugar levels after meals by up to 20-30%. Better still make an apple cider vinegar and olive oil dressing for your salad and eat that before your main meal.
- If you are eating good food but still experiencing high sugar levels try reducing your portion size.
- If particular foods were ok one day but caused a spike in your sugar levels on another day be aware of how other factors are impacting your day such as hydration, tiredness, stress or illness.

If you are stuck for what to eat, here are some ideas:

Breakfast
- Fish, eggs, or avocado on sourdough toast
- Frittata – add veg for extra nutrients
- Natural full fat Greek yoghurt with nuts/seeds, nut butter and berries

A note about porridge: Some people find they have high blood sugar after eating oats. Try reducing portion size and adding nut/seeds, nut butter, blueberries and a spoon of ghee or coconut oil whilst cooking. Use steel cut oats as they are less processed than rolled or instant oats.

Lunch
- Vegetable fritters with eggs, avocado and bacon
- Shakshuka with avocado and sourdough
- Sausages, broccoli or peas with sweet potato mash
- Chicken and tabbouleh quinoa salad
- Chicken tenders with cabbage slaw
- Roasted salmon with peppers, courgettes, tomatoes and sweet potato

Dinner
- Turkey meatballs with courgetti and butterbeans
- Chickpea curry, cottage cheese and steamed broccoli
- Fishcakes and steamed vegetables
- Chicken curry with cauliflower rice
- Kitchari made with lentils and buckwheat and side salad
- Steak, sweet potato fries and salad
- Tofu and kidney bean chickpea pancake with slaw

Snacks

- Apples and nut butter or cheese
- Carrots, peppers, cucumbers and humous
- Blueberries
- Nuts/seeds
- Cheese and oatcakes
- Slice of deli meat and cheese
- Rye bread topped with avocado
- Good quality 70% dark chocolate
- Bone broth

———————● TIPS ●———————

- Always have healthy snacks at hand, especially when you are travelling.
- Try eating potatoes cooled and not roasting hot. Once potatoes are cooled the sugar in the potatoes becomes resistant to human digestion and therefore there is less of a blood sugar spike.

CHAPTER 5

CRAVINGS

Pregnancy and cravings go hand in hand! It's inevitable. Below are some tips and alternatives to help keep you on track.

Carbohydrates

Bread
If you are craving bread find a good sourdough made with whole grains, check the ingredients, the good ones will only contain flour, starter, salt and water and that's it! If it's hard to come by, buy a couple of loaves, slice and pop them into the freezer so you have it to hand when you need it. Have the bread with something like avocado, peanut butter, cheese, eggs or meat. You could also give rye bread a try. Its denser and quite filling and you may tolerate it better than other breads.

Pasta
Have whole grain pasta, or you could even try chickpea, lentil or pea pasta and see if you get a different blood sugar response. Keep in mind the portion and how to plate up your food.

Wraps

A good wrap alternative is to make them at home using just chickpea flour and water. Chickpeas are higher in protein and lower in carbohydrates than wheat flour. You want a pancake batter type consistency and cook like you would a crepe. You can find recipes on YouTube by searching for 'chickpea flour tortillas recipe'.

Something sweet

Cakes/cookies

Make your own and reduce the amount of sugar and substitute flour with almond flour instead. You can also find recipes that use apples/bananas as a little sweetener instead of sugar. Batch make the dough and store in the freezer and bake when needed. Here are some links for ideas:

Banana bread:
https://detoxinista.com/almond-flour-banana-bread/

Cookies:
https://www.lazycatkitchen.com/vegan-almond-cookies/

Chocolate chip cookies:
https://downshiftology.com/recipes/gluten-free-chocolate-chip-cookies/#wprm-recipe-container-53142

Chocolate
Have a couple of squares of good quality dark chocolate (minimum 70% cocoa). Or you could try this avocado chocolate mousse, its full of good fats: https://downshiftology.com/recipes/chocolate-avocado-pudding/#wprm-recipe-container-33866

Chia pudding
This is both nutritious and satisfying. Chia seeds are rich in fibre, omega-3 fat and minerals. The chia seeds give the pudding like texture when soaked in liquid and you can use milk, coconut milk or any nut milk. Make it yourself, here's a recipe by Downshiftology: https://downshiftology.com/recipes/how-to-make-chia-seed-pudding/#wprm-recipe-container-32951

Make your own ice cream.
If you have the energy make some homemade ice cream but reduce the amount of sugar by 50%. I regularly make this classic BBC recipe using half of the sugar and I promise you it still tastes good! https://www.bbcgoodfood.com/recipes/ultimate-vanilla-ice-cream

Strawberries and cream
Yes! Strawberries have a low glycaemic index and paired with some double (heavy) cream it shouldn't make your blood sugars spike but watch your portions.

Salty/crunchy

Homemade crackers
Instead of reaching for the usual crisps or chips, give these homemade crackers made of seeds a go. Recipe by Downshiftology:
https://downshiftology.com/recipes/ultimate-seed-crackers/#wprm-recipe-container-32446

Lotus seeds
Roast some lotus seeds / foxnut and add spices/flavourings of choice. Lotus seeds are rich in nutrients and will give you the crunch you are craving.

Nut/seed mix
The classic nuts / seeds will often do the trick and are filling. Just check the labels first or roast your own.

——————————● TIPS ●——————————

A few other tactics to try when cravings hit:
- Have what you really want but reduce the portion size, a couple of bites might be enough to satisfy the craving. Then go for a short walk.

- Thoughtfully pair the food with other high protein or fatty foods. For example, have natural full fat Greek yoghurt, nuts/seeds, peanut butter with your cake/cookie. The combination of more protein/fat may reduce the sugar spike you would have had if you'd eaten the cake/cookie alone. It will also be more filling and nutritious.

CHAPTER 6

EXERCISE

You will want to incorporate exercise and movement into your daily routine. Not only will this help with stress management and sugar levels but with stamina during labour and afterwards when baby is here!

Check with your Healthcare Practitioner about what is safe for you before you embark on anything new.

Pre-natal yoga
Prenatal yoga is specifically designed for pregnant women and is a low impact safe way to incorporate exercise. It can help increase strength and flexibility, reduce stress, decrease aches and pains stretch, and help you sleep.

There may be classes local to you which you can attend and it's also a great way to make friends. If you need something convenient there are many online classes to try.

Walking

After a meal, within one hour of eating go for a 20-minute walk. It makes a big difference to your post meal reading. Test it a few times if you need convincing of the benefits – compare readings when you walk and don't walk and see for yourself!

As you get further along your pregnancy, it may become harder to control your blood sugar levels. You may also experience drop in energy levels making any kind of exercise difficult. Make sure you speak to your Healthcare Practitioner and follow their advice.

─────────● TIPS ●─────────

If it's raining or too cold outside, or you can't get out of the house because you have young children, search on YouTube for walking workouts or just put on some music and move around the house instead. 20 minutes of continuous gentle movement should do it.

CHAPTER 7

STRESS REDUCTION

You may have a busy family life, running around after young children, working, deadlines, a list as long as your arm of things to do before the baby arrives but you are going to want to find ways to reduce the stress in your life and find ways of managing it. When under stress, the body releases hormones that can cause blood sugar levels to increase.

Find out what is causing you to feel stressed and see if there are ways you can reduce or eliminate it.

TIPS

- As mentioned previously exercise can help, so try and get movement into your day.
- Make sure you rest when you need to and get a good night's sleep.
- Talking can help. Talk to friends, family or a professional if that helps.
- Ask for more help. Ask your partner to do more, ask grandparents to look after the kids, get a cleaner if possible.
- Do something that helps you relax like taking a warm bath, going for a walk, reading a good book or watching your favourite tv show.
- Try meditating and breathing exercises. You can find many guided meditations online.

CHAPTER 8

MEDICATION

Sometimes diet and exercise are not enough. If your blood sugar levels are not within target levels and you are struggling to stabilise them you may be given medicine. There are two options:

Metformin
Metformin lowers blood sugar levels by reducing how much glucose is released from the liver, and by helping the cells of your body to absorb more glucose from the bloodstream. This is a tablet and is taken up to three times a day, with or after a meal.

Insulin
You will most likely be prescribed insulin if your blood sugar levels are very high and if metformin does not work well enough. Insulin does need to be injected using an insulin pen. There are two types of insulin:

- A rapid acting insulin which is taken just before a meal. This insulin works for a shorter period of time (3-5 hours).
- Longer acting insulin which is only once a day.

Your Healthcare Practitioner will discuss the best type of insulin and dose for you and will show you how to inject. You will still need to keep testing your blood sugar levels.

You need to keep an eye out for high blood sugar (also known as hyperglycaemia). If your readings are high more than three times a week you may need more insulin. You will need to speak to your Healthcare Practitioner so they can adjust your medication. Keep in mind that you will become more insulin resistant as your pregnancy progresses, so you may need to keep increasing your dose.

Hypoglycaemia (low blood sugar) is when you blood sugar drops below 4 mmol/l or 70 mg/dL. It is important to be aware of the signs and symptoms of hypoglycaemia so you can act quickly if it does occur.

Signs/symptoms:
- Light headed, dizzy
- Irritable and/or confused
- Tired, hungry
- Can't see clearly

Follow the advice given to you by your Healthcare Practitioner. They will most likely tell you to eat or drink something sweet like fruit juice, a spoon of honey and check your blood sugar levels 15 minutes later.

CHAPTER 9

TRACK DAILY AND LEARN QUICKLY

Everyone is different and what works for one person will not work for another. There is a bit of trial and error needed here and that's why it's important to keep a detailed journal or diary. It will help you learn what works for you in terms of food, exercise and stress reduction. It will also help identify other factors that may be making your glucose levels high, for example sleep quality, fatigue, hydration levels. The quicker you learn, the quicker you'll be able to gain some control.

As you get closer to your due date, your sugar levels could become harder to control and what was working no longer does, you may want to speak to your Healthcare Practitioner at this point to get advice. Consider switching to smaller but more frequent meals.

BIRTH AND BEYOND

During your pregnancy you will have additional appointments with your Healthcare Practitioner. They will track the size of the baby, your blood sugar levels and discuss a birth plan.

Generally, it is recommended that baby is delivered by 40 weeks and you'll be scheduled for an induction if baby hasn't arrived by then.

It will be important to control your blood sugar levels during labour as it will help your baby have better blood sugar levels at birth. Once the baby is born and able to produce its own insulin there's a chance the baby could have low blood sugar. Your baby's blood sugars will be tested a few hours after birth and if all is ok, you'll be cleared to move to the ward or go home.

Your blood sugars will also need to be tested after birth. You should find that due to the hormone drop that your sugar levels return to normal shortly after birth. However, the timeframe for this will vary from person to person. You'll be tested again at 4-12 weeks and then every 1-3 years.

The future

Up to half of all women who had gestational diabetes go on to develop type 2 diabetes with 5 years of giving birth. It's important to continue with a balanced diet, regular exercise and looking after yourself.

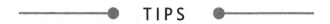 **TIPS**

- Pack plenty of snacks in your hospital bag. Hospitals don't always have suitable food available or may not cater for diabetic diet.

Personal note

As you conclude this exploration of gestational diabetes, take heart in the realization that amidst the challenges, there exists a tapestry of positivity. Your journey signifies not only resilience but also the promise of a healthy pregnancy and a vibrant future for both you and your baby.

Embrace the newfound strength and knowledge, and step into the next chapter of motherhood with confidence.

Here's to the beautiful balance of challenges and triumphs, leading to a future filled with joy, good health, and the enduring love that accompanies the miracle of life. Congratulations on navigating this path with grace and courage!

Useful resources

Follow us on Instagram for more advice, tips, tricks and hacks:
about_gestational_diabetes

NHS Gestational Diabetes:
https://www.nhs.uk/conditions/gestational-diabetes/

American Diabetes Association:
https://diabetes.org/about-diabetes/gestational-diabetes

National Institute of Diabetes and Digestive and Kidney Diseases:
https://www.niddk.nih.gov/health-information/diabetes/overview/what-is-diabetes/gestational

DATE:	FASTING	BREAKFAST		LUNCH		DINNER		BEDTIME
		PRE	POST	PRE	POST	PRE	POST	
MONDAY								
TUESDAY								
WEDNESDAY								
THURSDAY								
FRIDAY								
SATURDAY								
SUNDAY								

DATE:	FASTING	BREAKFAST		LUNCH		DINNER		BEDTIME
		PRE	POST	PRE	POST	PRE	POST	
MONDAY								
TUESDAY								
WEDNESDAY								
THURSDAY								
FRIDAY								
SATURDAY								
SUNDAY								

DATE:	FASTING	BREAKFAST		LUNCH		DINNER		BEDTIME
		PRE	POST	PRE	POST	PRE	POST	
MONDAY								
TUESDAY								
WEDNESDAY								
THURSDAY								
FRIDAY								
SATURDAY								
SUNDAY								

DATE:	FASTING	BREAKFAST		LUNCH		DINNER		BEDTIME
		PRE	POST	PRE	POST	PRE	POST	
MONDAY								
TUESDAY								
WEDNESDAY								
THURSDAY								
FRIDAY								
SATURDAY								
SUNDAY								

DATE:	FASTING	BREAKFAST		LUNCH		DINNER		BEDTIME
		PRE	POST	PRE	POST	PRE	POST	
MONDAY								
TUESDAY								
WEDNESDAY								
THURSDAY								
FRIDAY								
SATURDAY								
SUNDAY								

DATE:	FASTING	BREAKFAST		LUNCH		DINNER		BEDTIME
		PRE	POST	PRE	POST	PRE	POST	
MONDAY								
TUESDAY								
WEDNESDAY								
THURSDAY								
FRIDAY								
SATURDAY								
SUNDAY								

DATE:	FASTING	BREAKFAST		LUNCH		DINNER		BEDTIME
		PRE	POST	PRE	POST	PRE	POST	
MONDAY								
TUESDAY								
WEDNESDAY								
THURSDAY								
FRIDAY								
SATURDAY								
SUNDAY								

DATE:	FASTING	BREAKFAST		LUNCH		DINNER		BEDTIME
		PRE	POST	PRE	POST	PRE	POST	
MONDAY								
TUESDAY								
WEDNESDAY								
THURSDAY								
FRIDAY								
SATURDAY								
SUNDAY								

DATE:	FASTING	BREAKFAST		LUNCH		DINNER		BEDTIME
		PRE	POST	PRE	POST	PRE	POST	
MONDAY								
TUESDAY								
WEDNESDAY								
THURSDAY								
FRIDAY								
SATURDAY								
SUNDAY								

DATE:	FASTING	BREAKFAST		LUNCH		DINNER		BEDTIME
		PRE	POST	PRE	POST	PRE	POST	
MONDAY								
TUESDAY								
WEDNESDAY								
THURSDAY								
FRIDAY								
SATURDAY								
SUNDAY								

DATE:	FASTING	BREAKFAST		LUNCH		DINNER		BEDTIME
		PRE	POST	PRE	POST	PRE	POST	
MONDAY								
TUESDAY								
WEDNESDAY								
THURSDAY								
FRIDAY								
SATURDAY								
SUNDAY								

DATE:	FASTING	BREAKFAST		LUNCH		DINNER		BEDTIME
		PRE	POST	PRE	POST	PRE	POST	
MONDAY								
TUESDAY								
WEDNESDAY								
THURSDAY								
FRIDAY								
SATURDAY								
SUNDAY								

DATE:	FASTING	BREAKFAST		LUNCH		DINNER		BEDTIME
		PRE	POST	PRE	POST	PRE	POST	
MONDAY								
TUESDAY								
WEDNESDAY								
THURSDAY								
FRIDAY								
SATURDAY								
SUNDAY								

DATE:	FASTING	BREAKFAST		LUNCH		DINNER		BEDTIME
		PRE	POST	PRE	POST	PRE	POST	
MONDAY								
TUESDAY								
WEDNESDAY								
THURSDAY								
FRIDAY								
SATURDAY								
SUNDAY								

DATE:	FASTING	BREAKFAST		LUNCH		DINNER		BEDTIME
		PRE	POST	PRE	POST	PRE	POST	
MONDAY								
TUESDAY								
WEDNESDAY								
THURSDAY								
FRIDAY								
SATURDAY								
SUNDAY								

DATE:	FASTING	BREAKFAST		LUNCH		DINNER		BEDTIME
		PRE	POST	PRE	POST	PRE	POST	
MONDAY								
TUESDAY								
WEDNESDAY								
THURSDAY								
FRIDAY								
SATURDAY								
SUNDAY								

M / T / W / T / F / S / S   DATE:

Meal	Blood sugar levels		Notes
	PRE	POST	
FASTING	TIME:		
BREAKFAST	TIME:	TIME:	
LUNCH	TIME:	TIME:	
DINNER	TIME:	TIME:	
SNACKS			

WEIGHT:

EXERCISE:

SLEEP QUALITY: POOR / OK / GOOD / GREAT

STRESS LEVELS: NONE / LOW / MEDIUM / HIGH

HYDRATION: ▢ ▢ ▢ ▢ ▢ ▢ ▢ ▢

M / T / W / T / F / S / S   DATE:

Meal	Blood sugar levels		Notes
FASTING	TIME:		
	PRE	POST	
BREAKFAST	TIME:	TIME:	
LUNCH	TIME:	TIME:	
DINNER	TIME:	TIME:	
SNACKS	TIME:		
WEIGHT:			
EXERCISE:			

SLEEP QUALITY: POOR / OK / GOOD / GREAT

STRESS LEVELS: NONE / LOW / MEDIUM / HIGH

HYDRATION: ☐ ☐ ☐ ☐ ☐ ☐ ☐ ☐

Meal	Blood sugar levels		Notes
	PRE	POST	
FASTING	TIME:		
BREAKFAST	TIME:	TIME:	
LUNCH	TIME:	TIME:	
DINNER	TIME:	TIME:	
SNACKS	TIME:		

SLEEP QUALITY: POOR / OK / GOOD / GREAT   WEIGHT:

STRESS LEVELS: NONE / LOW / MEDIUM / HIGH   EXERCISE:

HYDRATION: ☐ ☐ ☐ ☐ ☐ ☐ ☐ ☐

M / T / W / T / F / S / S   DATE:

Meal	Blood sugar levels		Notes
	TIME:		
FASTING			
	PRE	POST	
BREAKFAST	TIME:	TIME:	
LUNCH	TIME:	TIME:	
DINNER	TIME:	TIME:	
SNACKS			
	WEIGHT:		
	EXERCISE:		

SLEEP QUALITY: POOR / OK / GOOD / GREAT

STRESS LEVELS: NONE / LOW / MEDIUM / HIGH

HYDRATION: ▢ ▢ ▢ ▢ ▢ ▢ ▢

M / T / W / T / F / S / S   DATE:

Meal	Blood sugar levels		Notes
FASTING	TIME:		
BREAKFAST	PRE TIME:	POST TIME:	
LUNCH	TIME:	TIME:	
DINNER	TIME:	TIME:	
SNACKS			

WEIGHT:

EXERCISE:

SLEEP QUALITY: POOR / OK / GOOD / GREAT

STRESS LEVELS: NONE / LOW / MEDIUM / HIGH

HYDRATION: ▢ ▢ ▢ ▢ ▢ ▢ ▢ ▢

M / T / W / T / F / S / S   DATE:

Meal	Blood sugar levels		Notes
FASTING	TIME:		
BREAKFAST	PRE TIME:	POST TIME:	
LUNCH	TIME:	TIME:	
DINNER	TIME:	TIME:	
SNACKS			

WEIGHT:

EXERCISE:

SLEEP QUALITY: POOR / OK / GOOD / GREAT

STRESS LEVELS: NONE / LOW / MEDIUM / HIGH

HYDRATION: ☐ ☐ ☐ ☐ ☐ ☐ ☐ ☐

M / T / W / T / F / S / S   DATE:

Meal	Blood sugar levels		Notes
FASTING	TIME:		
	PRE	POST	
BREAKFAST	TIME:	TIME:	
LUNCH	TIME:	TIME:	
DINNER	TIME:	TIME:	
SNACKS	TIME:		

WEIGHT:

EXERCISE:

SLEEP QUALITY: POOR / OK / GOOD / GREAT

STRESS LEVELS: NONE / LOW / MEDIUM / HIGH

HYDRATION: ▢ ▢ ▢ ▢ ▢ ▢ ▢ ▢

M / T / W / T / F / S / S   DATE:

Meal	Blood sugar levels		Notes
FASTING	TIME:		
	PRE	POST	
BREAKFAST	TIME:	TIME:	
LUNCH	TIME:	TIME:	
DINNER	TIME:	TIME:	
SNACKS	TIME:		

WEIGHT:

EXERCISE:

SLEEP QUALITY: POOR / OK / GOOD / GREAT

STRESS LEVELS: NONE / LOW / MEDIUM / HIGH

HYDRATION: ☐ ☐ ☐ ☐ ☐ ☐ ☐ ☐

M / T / W / T / F / S / S   DATE:

Meal	Blood sugar levels		Notes
	PRE	POST	
FASTING	TIME:		
BREAKFAST	TIME:	TIME:	
LUNCH	TIME:	TIME:	
DINNER	TIME:	TIME:	
SNACKS			

WEIGHT:

EXERCISE:

SLEEP QUALITY: POOR / OK / GOOD / GREAT

STRESS LEVELS: NONE / LOW / MEDIUM / HIGH

HYDRATION: ☐ ☐ ☐ ☐ ☐ ☐ ☐ ☐

M / T / W / T / F / S / S   DATE:

Meal	Blood sugar levels		Notes
	PRE	POST	
FASTING	TIME:		
BREAKFAST	TIME:	TIME:	
LUNCH	TIME:	TIME:	
DINNER	TIME:	TIME:	
SNACKS			

WEIGHT:

EXERCISE:

SLEEP QUALITY: POOR / OK / GOOD / GREAT

STRESS LEVELS: NONE / LOW / MEDIUM / HIGH

HYDRATION: ☐ ☐ ☐ ☐ ☐ ☐ ☐

M / T / W / T / F / S / S   DATE:

Meal	Blood sugar levels		Notes
FASTING	TIME:		
BREAKFAST	PRE	POST	
	TIME:	TIME:	
LUNCH	TIME:	TIME:	
DINNER	TIME:	TIME:	
SNACKS			

WEIGHT:

EXERCISE:

SLEEP QUALITY: POOR / OK / GOOD / GREAT

STRESS LEVELS: NONE / LOW / MEDIUM / HIGH

HYDRATION: ▢ ▢ ▢ ▢ ▢ ▢ ▢ ▢

M / T / W / T / F / S / S   DATE:

Meal	Blood sugar levels		Notes
	PRE	POST	
FASTING	TIME:		
BREAKFAST	TIME:	TIME:	
LUNCH	TIME:	TIME:	
DINNER	TIME:	TIME:	
SNACKS			

SLEEP QUALITY: POOR / OK / GOOD / GREAT

STRESS LEVELS: NONE / LOW / MEDIUM / HIGH

HYDRATION: ☐ ☐ ☐ ☐ ☐ ☐ ☐ ☐

WEIGHT:

EXERCISE:

M / T / W / T / F / S / S   DATE:

Meal	Blood sugar levels		Notes
	TIME:		
	PRE	POST	
FASTING			
BREAKFAST	TIME:	TIME:	
LUNCH	TIME:	TIME:	
DINNER	TIME:	TIME:	
SNACKS	TIME:		

WEIGHT:

EXERCISE:

SLEEP QUALITY: POOR / OK / GOOD / GREAT

STRESS LEVELS: NONE / LOW / MEDIUM / HIGH

HYDRATION: ☐ ☐ ☐ ☐ ☐ ☐ ☐ ☐

M / T / W / T / F / S / S   DATE:

Meal	Blood sugar levels		Notes
FASTING	TIME:		
BREAKFAST	PRE TIME:	POST TIME:	
LUNCH	TIME:	TIME:	
DINNER	TIME:	TIME:	
SNACKS	TIME:		

WEIGHT:

EXERCISE:

SLEEP QUALITY: POOR / OK / GOOD / GREAT

STRESS LEVELS: NONE / LOW / MEDIUM / HIGH

HYDRATION: ☐☐☐☐☐☐☐☐

M / T / W / T / F / S / S   DATE:

Meal	Blood sugar levels		Notes
	TIME:		
FASTING			
	PRE	POST	
		TIME:	
BREAKFAST			
	TIME:	TIME:	
LUNCH			
	TIME:	TIME:	
DINNER			
	TIME:		
SNACKS			

WEIGHT:

EXERCISE:

SLEEP QUALITY: POOR / OK / GOOD / GREAT

STRESS LEVELS: NONE / LOW / MEDIUM / HIGH

HYDRATION: ☐ ☐ ☐ ☐ ☐ ☐ ☐ ☐

M / T / W / T / F / S / S   DATE:

Meal	Blood sugar levels		Notes
	TIME:		
	PRE	POST	
FASTING	TIME:		
BREAKFAST	TIME:	TIME:	
LUNCH	TIME:	TIME:	
DINNER	TIME:	TIME:	
SNACKS			

WEIGHT:

EXERCISE:

SLEEP QUALITY: POOR / OK / GOOD / GREAT

STRESS LEVELS: NONE / LOW / MEDIUM / HIGH

HYDRATION: ☐ ☐ ☐ ☐ ☐ ☐ ☐ ☐

M / T / W / T / F / S / S   DATE:

Meal	Blood sugar levels		Notes
FASTING	TIME:		
	PRE	POST	
BREAKFAST	TIME:	TIME:	
LUNCH	TIME:	TIME:	
DINNER	TIME:	TIME:	
SNACKS	TIME:	TIME:	

WEIGHT:

EXERCISE:

SLEEP QUALITY: POOR / OK / GOOD / GREAT

STRESS LEVELS: NONE / LOW / MEDIUM / HIGH

HYDRATION: ▢ ▢ ▢ ▢ ▢ ▢ ▢ ▢

M / T / W / T / F / S / S   DATE:

Meal	Blood sugar levels		Notes
FASTING	TIME:		
BREAKFAST	PRE TIME:	POST TIME:	
LUNCH	TIME:	TIME:	
DINNER	TIME:	TIME:	
SNACKS			

WEIGHT:

EXERCISE:

SLEEP QUALITY: POOR / OK / GOOD / GREAT

STRESS LEVELS: NONE / LOW / MEDIUM / HIGH

HYDRATION: ☐ ☐ ☐ ☐ ☐ ☐

M / T / W / T / F / S / S   DATE:

Meal	Blood sugar levels		Notes
	PRE	POST	
FASTING	TIME:		
BREAKFAST	TIME:	TIME:	
LUNCH	TIME:	TIME:	
DINNER	TIME:	TIME:	
SNACKS	TIME:		

WEIGHT:

EXERCISE:

SLEEP QUALITY: POOR / OK / GOOD / GREAT

STRESS LEVELS: NONE / LOW / MEDIUM / HIGH

HYDRATION: ☐☐☐☐☐ ☐☐☐

M / T / W / T / F / S / S   DATE:

Meal	Blood sugar levels		Notes
FASTING	TIME:		
BREAKFAST	PRE TIME:	POST TIME:	
LUNCH	TIME:	TIME:	
DINNER	TIME:	TIME:	
SNACKS	TIME:		

WEIGHT:

EXERCISE:

SLEEP QUALITY: POOR / OK / GOOD / GREAT

STRESS LEVELS: NONE / LOW / MEDIUM / HIGH

HYDRATION: ☐ ☐ ☐ ☐ ☐ ☐ ☐

M / T / W / T / F / S / S   DATE:

Meal	Blood sugar levels		Notes
FASTING	TIME:		
	PRE	POST	
BREAKFAST	TIME:	TIME:	
LUNCH	TIME:	TIME:	
DINNER	TIME:	TIME:	
SNACKS	TIME:		

WEIGHT:

EXERCISE:

SLEEP QUALITY: POOR / OK / GOOD / GREAT

STRESS LEVELS: NONE / LOW / MEDIUM / HIGH

HYDRATION: ▢ ▢ ▢ ▢ ▢ ▢ ▢ ▢

M / T / W / T / F / S / S   DATE:

Meal	Blood sugar levels		Notes
FASTING	TIME:		
BREAKFAST	PRE TIME:	POST TIME:	
LUNCH	TIME:	TIME:	
DINNER	TIME:	TIME:	
SNACKS	TIME:		

WEIGHT:

EXERCISE:

SLEEP QUALITY: POOR / OK / GOOD / GREAT

STRESS LEVELS: NONE / LOW / MEDIUM / HIGH

HYDRATION: ▯ ▯ ▯ ▯ ▯ ▯ ▯

M / T / W / T / F / S / S   DATE:

Meal	Blood sugar levels		Notes
FASTING	TIME:		
	PRE	POST	
BREAKFAST	TIME:	TIME:	
LUNCH	TIME:	TIME:	
DINNER	TIME:	TIME:	
SNACKS	TIME:		

WEIGHT:

EXERCISE:

SLEEP QUALITY: POOR / OK / GOOD / GREAT

STRESS LEVELS: NONE / LOW / MEDIUM / HIGH

HYDRATION: ☐ ☐ ☐ ☐ ☐ ☐ ☐

M / T / W / T / F / S / S   DATE:

Meal	Blood sugar levels		Notes
FASTING	TIME:		
BREAKFAST	PRE TIME:	POST TIME:	
LUNCH	TIME:	TIME:	
DINNER	TIME:	TIME:	
SNACKS			

WEIGHT:

EXERCISE:

SLEEP QUALITY: POOR / OK / GOOD / GREAT

STRESS LEVELS: NONE / LOW / MEDIUM / HIGH

HYDRATION: ☐ ☐ ☐ ☐ ☐ ☐ ☐

M / T / W / T / F / S / S   DATE:

Meal	Blood sugar levels		Notes
FASTING	TIME:		
	PRE	POST	
BREAKFAST	TIME:	TIME:	
LUNCH	TIME:	TIME:	
DINNER	TIME:	TIME:	
SNACKS	TIME:		

SLEEP QUALITY: POOR / OK / GOOD / GREAT   WEIGHT:

STRESS LEVELS: NONE / LOW / MEDIUM / HIGH   EXERCISE:

HYDRATION: ☐ ☐ ☐ ☐ ☐ ☐ ☐ ☐

M / T / W / T / F / S / S   DATE:

Meal	Blood sugar levels		Notes
	PRE	POST	
FASTING	TIME:		
BREAKFAST	TIME:	TIME:	
LUNCH	TIME:	TIME:	
DINNER	TIME:	TIME:	
SNACKS	TIME:		

WEIGHT:

EXERCISE:

SLEEP QUALITY: POOR / OK / GOOD / GREAT

STRESS LEVELS: NONE / LOW / MEDIUM / HIGH

HYDRATION: ▢ ▢ ▢ ▢ ▢ ▢ ▢ ▢

M / T / W / T / F / S / S   DATE:

Meal	Blood sugar levels		Notes
FASTING	TIME:		
BREAKFAST	PRE	POST	
	TIME:	TIME:	
LUNCH	TIME:	TIME:	
DINNER	TIME:	TIME:	
SNACKS			

WEIGHT:

EXERCISE:

SLEEP QUALITY: POOR / OK / GOOD / GREAT

STRESS LEVELS: NONE / LOW / MEDIUM / HIGH

HYDRATION: ☐ ☐ ☐ ☐ ☐ ☐ ☐ ☐

M / T / W / T / F / S / S   DATE:

Meal	Blood sugar levels		Notes
FASTING	TIME:		
BREAKFAST	PRE TIME:	POST TIME:	
LUNCH	TIME:		
DINNER	TIME:		
SNACKS	TIME:		

WEIGHT:

EXERCISE:

SLEEP QUALITY: POOR / OK / GOOD / GREAT

STRESS LEVELS: NONE / LOW / MEDIUM / HIGH

HYDRATION: ☐ ☐ ☐ ☐ ☐ ☐ ☐ ☐ ☐

M / T / W / T / F / S / S   DATE:

Meal	Blood sugar levels		Notes
	PRE	POST	
FASTING	TIME:		
BREAKFAST	TIME:	TIME:	
LUNCH	TIME:	TIME:	
DINNER	TIME:	TIME:	
SNACKS			

WEIGHT:

EXERCISE:

SLEEP QUALITY: POOR / OK / GOOD / GREAT

STRESS LEVELS: NONE / LOW / MEDIUM / HIGH

HYDRATION: ☐ ☐ ☐ ☐ ☐ ☐ ☐ ☐

M / T / W / T / F / S / S   DATE:

Meal	Blood sugar levels		Notes
FASTING	TIME:		
BREAKFAST	PRE	POST	
	TIME:	TIME:	
LUNCH	TIME:	TIME:	
DINNER	TIME:	TIME:	
SNACKS			

WEIGHT:

EXERCISE:

SLEEP QUALITY: POOR / OK / GOOD / GREAT

STRESS LEVELS: NONE / LOW / MEDIUM / HIGH

HYDRATION: ☐ ☐ ☐ ☐ ☐ ☐ ☐ ☐

M / T / W / T / F / S / S   DATE:

Meal	Blood sugar levels		Notes
	TIME:		
	PRE	POST	
FASTING	TIME:	TIME:	
BREAKFAST			
LUNCH	TIME:	TIME:	
DINNER	TIME:	TIME:	
SNACKS			

SLEEP QUALITY: POOR / OK / GOOD / GREAT

STRESS LEVELS: NONE / LOW / MEDIUM / HIGH

HYDRATION: ▢ ▢ ▢ ▢ ▢ ▢ ▢ ▢

WEIGHT:

EXERCISE:

M / T / W / T / F / S / S   DATE:

Meal	Blood sugar levels		Notes
	PRE	**POST**	
FASTING	TIME:		
BREAKFAST	TIME:	TIME:	
LUNCH	TIME:	TIME:	
DINNER	TIME:	TIME:	
SNACKS	TIME:		

WEIGHT:

EXERCISE:

SLEEP QUALITY: POOR / OK / GOOD / GREAT

STRESS LEVELS: NONE / LOW / MEDIUM / HIGH

HYDRATION: ▢ ▢ ▢ ▢ ▢ ▢ ▢

M / T / W / T / F / S / S   DATE:

Meal	Blood sugar levels		Notes
	TIME:		
FASTING			
	PRE	POST	
BREAKFAST	TIME:	TIME:	
LUNCH	TIME:	TIME:	
DINNER	TIME:	TIME:	
SNACKS	TIME:		

WEIGHT:

EXERCISE:

SLEEP QUALITY: POOR / OK / GOOD / GREAT

STRESS LEVELS: NONE / LOW / MEDIUM / HIGH

HYDRATION: ☐ ☐ ☐ ☐ ☐ ☐ ☐ ☐

M / T / W / T / F / S / S   DATE:

Meal	Blood sugar levels		Notes
FASTING	TIME:		
BREAKFAST	PRE TIME:	POST TIME:	
LUNCH	TIME:	TIME:	
DINNER	TIME:	TIME:	
SNACKS			

WEIGHT:

EXERCISE:

SLEEP QUALITY: POOR / OK / GOOD / GREAT

STRESS LEVELS: NONE / LOW / MEDIUM / HIGH

HYDRATION: ☐ ☐ ☐ ☐ ☐ ☐ ☐ ☐

M / T / W / T / F / S / S   DATE:

Meal	Blood sugar levels		Notes
	TIME:		
FASTING	PRE	POST	
BREAKFAST	TIME:	TIME:	
LUNCH	TIME:	TIME:	
DINNER	TIME:	TIME:	
SNACKS			

WEIGHT:

SLEEP QUALITY: POOR / OK / GOOD / GREAT

STRESS LEVELS: NONE / LOW / MEDIUM / HIGH

EXERCISE:

HYDRATION: ☐ ☐ ☐ ☐ ☐ ☐ ☐ ☐

M / T / W / T / F / S / S   DATE:

Meal	Blood sugar levels		Notes
	TIME:		
FASTING			
	PRE	POST	
BREAKFAST	TIME:	TIME:	
LUNCH	TIME:	TIME:	
DINNER	TIME:	TIME:	
SNACKS			

WEIGHT:

EXERCISE:

SLEEP QUALITY: POOR / OK / GOOD / GREAT

STRESS LEVELS: NONE / LOW / MEDIUM / HIGH

HYDRATION: ☐ ☐ ☐ ☐ ☐ ☐ ☐

M / T / W / T / F / S / S   DATE:

Meal	Blood sugar levels		Notes
	PRE	POST	
FASTING	TIME:		
BREAKFAST	TIME:	TIME:	
LUNCH	TIME:	TIME:	
DINNER	TIME:	TIME:	
SNACKS	TIME:		

WEIGHT:

EXERCISE:

SLEEP QUALITY: POOR / OK / GOOD / GREAT

STRESS LEVELS: NONE / LOW / MEDIUM / HIGH

HYDRATION: ☐ ☐ ☐ ☐ ☐ ☐ ☐ ☐

M / T / W / T / F / S / S   DATE:

Meal	Blood sugar levels		Notes
FASTING	TIME:		
	PRE	POST	
BREAKFAST	TIME:	TIME:	
LUNCH	TIME:	TIME:	
DINNER	TIME:	TIME:	
SNACKS			
	WEIGHT:		
	EXERCISE:		

SLEEP QUALITY: POOR / OK / GOOD / GREAT

STRESS LEVELS: NONE / LOW / MEDIUM / HIGH

HYDRATION: ▢ ▢ ▢ ▢ ▢ ▢ ▢ ▢

M / T / W / T / F / S / S   DATE:

Meal	Blood sugar levels		Notes
FASTING	TIME:		
BREAKFAST	PRE	POST	
	TIME:	TIME:	
LUNCH	TIME:	TIME:	
DINNER	TIME:	TIME:	
SNACKS	TIME:		

WEIGHT:

EXERCISE:

SLEEP QUALITY: POOR / OK / GOOD / GREAT

STRESS LEVELS: NONE / LOW / MEDIUM / HIGH

HYDRATION: ☐ ☐ ☐ ☐ ☐ ☐ ☐ ☐

M / T / W / T / F / S / S   DATE:

Meal	Blood sugar levels		Notes
FASTING	TIME:		
BREAKFAST	PRE TIME:	POST TIME:	
LUNCH	TIME:	TIME:	
DINNER	TIME:	TIME:	
SNACKS			

WEIGHT:

EXERCISE:

SLEEP QUALITY: POOR / OK / GOOD / GREAT

STRESS LEVELS: NONE / LOW / MEDIUM / HIGH

HYDRATION: ☐ ☐ ☐ ☐ ☐ ☐ ☐

M / T / W / T / F / S / S   DATE:

Meal	Blood sugar levels			Notes
FASTING	TIME:			
BREAKFAST	PRE TIME:	POST TIME:		
LUNCH	TIME:			
DINNER	TIME:			
SNACKS				

WEIGHT:

EXERCISE:

SLEEP QUALITY: POOR / OK / GOOD / GREAT

STRESS LEVELS: NONE / LOW / MEDIUM / HIGH

HYDRATION: ⬚ ⬚ ⬚ ⬚ ⬚ ⬚ ⬚ ⬚

M / T / W / T / F / S / S   DATE:

Meal	Blood sugar levels		Notes
	PRE	POST	
FASTING	TIME:		
BREAKFAST	TIME:	TIME:	
LUNCH	TIME:	TIME:	
DINNER	TIME:	TIME:	
SNACKS			

WEIGHT:

EXERCISE:

SLEEP QUALITY: POOR / OK / GOOD / GREAT

STRESS LEVELS: NONE / LOW / MEDIUM / HIGH

HYDRATION: ☐ ☐ ☐ ☐ ☐ ☐ ☐

M / T / W / T / F / S / S   DATE:

Meal	Blood sugar levels		Notes
FASTING	TIME:		
	PRE	POST	
BREAKFAST	TIME:	TIME:	
LUNCH	TIME:	TIME:	
DINNER	TIME:	TIME:	
SNACKS			

WEIGHT:

EXERCISE:

SLEEP QUALITY: POOR / OK / GOOD / GREAT

STRESS LEVELS: NONE / LOW / MEDIUM / HIGH

HYDRATION: ☐ ☐ ☐ ☐ ☐ ☐

M / T / W / T / F / S / S   DATE:

Meal	Blood sugar levels		Notes
	TIME:		
FASTING			
	PRE	POST	
BREAKFAST	TIME:	TIME:	
LUNCH	TIME:	TIME:	
DINNER	TIME:	TIME:	
SNACKS			

WEIGHT:

EXERCISE:

SLEEP QUALITY: POOR / OK / GOOD / GREAT

STRESS LEVELS: NONE / LOW / MEDIUM / HIGH

HYDRATION: ▢▢▢▢▢▢▢▢

M / T / W / T / F / S / S   DATE:

Meal	Blood sugar levels		Notes
FASTING	TIME:		
BREAKFAST	PRE TIME:	POST TIME:	
LUNCH	TIME:	TIME:	
DINNER	TIME:	TIME:	
SNACKS			

WEIGHT:

EXERCISE:

SLEEP QUALITY: POOR / OK / GOOD / GREAT

STRESS LEVELS: NONE / LOW / MEDIUM / HIGH

HYDRATION: ☐ ☐ ☐ ☐ ☐ ☐ ☐ ☐

M / T / W / T / F / S / S   DATE:

Meal	Blood sugar levels		Notes
	PRE	POST	
FASTING	TIME:		
BREAKFAST	TIME:	TIME:	
LUNCH	TIME:	TIME:	
DINNER	TIME:	TIME:	
SNACKS			

WEIGHT:

EXERCISE:

SLEEP QUALITY: POOR / OK / GOOD / GREAT

STRESS LEVELS: NONE / LOW / MEDIUM / HIGH

HYDRATION: ☐ ☐ ☐ ☐ ☐ ☐ ☐ ☐

M / T / W / T / F / S / S   DATE:

Meal	Blood sugar levels		Notes
	PRE	POST	
FASTING	TIME:		
BREAKFAST	TIME:	TIME:	
LUNCH	TIME:	TIME:	
DINNER	TIME:	TIME:	
SNACKS			

WEIGHT:

EXERCISE:

SLEEP QUALITY: POOR / OK / GOOD / GREAT

STRESS LEVELS: NONE / LOW / MEDIUM / HIGH

HYDRATION: ☐ ☐ ☐ ☐ ☐ ☐ ☐ ☐

M / T / W / T / F / S / S   DATE:

Meal	Blood sugar levels		Notes
FASTING	TIME:		
	PRE	POST	
BREAKFAST	TIME:	TIME:	
LUNCH	TIME:	TIME:	
DINNER	TIME:	TIME:	
SNACKS			

WEIGHT:

EXERCISE:

SLEEP QUALITY: POOR / OK / GOOD / GREAT

STRESS LEVELS: NONE / LOW / MEDIUM / HIGH

HYDRATION: ▢ ▢ ▢ ▢ ▢ ▢ ▢ ▢

M / T / W / T / F / S / S   DATE:

Meal	Blood sugar levels		Notes
FASTING	TIME:		
	PRE	POST	
BREAKFAST	TIME:	TIME:	
LUNCH	TIME:	TIME:	
DINNER	TIME:	TIME:	
SNACKS			

WEIGHT:

EXERCISE:

SLEEP QUALITY: POOR / OK / GOOD / GREAT

STRESS LEVELS: NONE / LOW / MEDIUM / HIGH

HYDRATION: ☐ ☐ ☐ ☐ ☐ ☐

M / T / W / T / F / S / S   DATE:

Meal	Blood sugar levels		Notes
FASTING	TIME:		
	PRE	POST	
BREAKFAST	TIME:	TIME:	
LUNCH	TIME:	TIME:	
DINNER	TIME:	TIME:	
SNACKS			

WEIGHT:

EXERCISE:

SLEEP QUALITY: POOR / OK / GOOD / GREAT

STRESS LEVELS: NONE / LOW / MEDIUM / HIGH

HYDRATION: ☐ ☐ ☐ ☐ ☐ ☐ ☐

M / T / W / T / F / S / S   DATE:

Meal	Blood sugar levels		Notes
	TIME:		
	PRE	POST	
FASTING	TIME:		
BREAKFAST	TIME:	TIME:	
LUNCH	TIME:	TIME:	
DINNER	TIME:	TIME:	
SNACKS			

SLEEP QUALITY: POOR / OK / GOOD / GREAT   WEIGHT:

STRESS LEVELS: NONE / LOW / MEDIUM / HIGH   EXERCISE:

HYDRATION: ☐ ☐ ☐ ☐ ☐ ☐

M / T / W / T / F / S / S   DATE:

Meal	Blood sugar levels		Notes
FASTING	TIME:		
	PRE	POST	
BREAKFAST	TIME:	TIME:	
LUNCH	TIME:	TIME:	
DINNER	TIME:	TIME:	
SNACKS	TIME:		
	WEIGHT:		
	EXERCISE:		

SLEEP QUALITY: POOR / OK / GOOD / GREAT

STRESS LEVELS: NONE / LOW / MEDIUM / HIGH

HYDRATION: ☐ ☐ ☐ ☐ ☐ ☐ ☐ ☐

M / T / W / T / F / S / S   DATE:

Meal	Blood sugar levels		Notes
	TIME:		
	PRE	POST	
FASTING			
BREAKFAST	TIME:	TIME:	
LUNCH	TIME:	TIME:	
DINNER	TIME:	TIME:	
SNACKS			

WEIGHT:

EXERCISE:

SLEEP QUALITY: POOR / OK / GOOD / GREAT

STRESS LEVELS: NONE / LOW / MEDIUM / HIGH

HYDRATION: ☐ ☐ ☐ ☐ ☐ ☐ ☐ ☐

M / T / W / T / F / S / S   DATE:

Meal	Blood sugar levels		Notes
	TIME:		
FASTING			
	PRE	POST	
BREAKFAST	TIME:	TIME:	
LUNCH	TIME:	TIME:	
DINNER	TIME:	TIME:	
SNACKS			

WEIGHT:

EXERCISE:

SLEEP QUALITY: POOR / OK / GOOD / GREAT

STRESS LEVELS: NONE / LOW / MEDIUM / HIGH

HYDRATION: ▢ ▢ ▢ ▢ ▢ ▢ ▢ ▢

M / T / W / T / F / S / S   DATE:

Meal	Blood sugar levels		Notes
	TIME:		
	PRE	POST	
BREAKFAST	TIME:	TIME:	
LUNCH	TIME:	TIME:	
DINNER	TIME:	TIME:	
SNACKS			

FASTING

SLEEP QUALITY: POOR / OK / GOOD / GREAT

STRESS LEVELS: NONE / LOW / MEDIUM / HIGH

HYDRATION: ☐ ☐ ☐ ☐ ☐ ☐ ☐ ☐

WEIGHT:

EXERCISE:

M / T / W / T / F / S / S   DATE:

Meal	Blood sugar levels		Notes
FASTING	TIME:		
	PRE	POST	
BREAKFAST	TIME:	TIME:	
LUNCH	TIME:	TIME:	
DINNER	TIME:	TIME:	
SNACKS	TIME:		
WEIGHT:			
EXERCISE:			

SLEEP QUALITY: POOR / OK / GOOD / GREAT

STRESS LEVELS: NONE / LOW / MEDIUM / HIGH

HYDRATION: ▢ ▢ ▢ ▢ ▢ ▢ ▢ ▢

M / T / W / T / F / S / S   DATE:

Meal	Blood sugar levels		Notes
	TIME:		
FASTING			
	PRE	POST	
	TIME:	TIME:	
BREAKFAST			
	TIME:	TIME:	
LUNCH			
	TIME:	TIME:	
DINNER			
	TIME:		
SNACKS			

WEIGHT:

EXERCISE:

SLEEP QUALITY: POOR / OK / GOOD / GREAT

STRESS LEVELS: NONE / LOW / MEDIUM / HIGH

HYDRATION: ☐ ☐ ☐ ☐ ☐ ☐ ☐ ☐

M / T / W / T / F / S / S   DATE:

Meal	Blood sugar levels		Notes
	TIME:		
	PRE	POST	
FASTING			
BREAKFAST	TIME:	TIME:	
LUNCH	TIME:	TIME:	
DINNER	TIME:	TIME:	
SNACKS			

WEIGHT:

EXERCISE:

SLEEP QUALITY: POOR / OK / GOOD / GREAT

STRESS LEVELS: NONE / LOW / MEDIUM / HIGH

HYDRATION: ☐ ☐ ☐ ☐ ☐ ☐ ☐

M / T / W / T / F / S / S   DATE:

Meal	Blood sugar levels		Notes
	PRE	POST	
FASTING	TIME:		
BREAKFAST	TIME:	TIME:	
LUNCH	TIME:	TIME:	
DINNER	TIME:	TIME:	
SNACKS	TIME:	TIME:	

WEIGHT:

EXERCISE:

SLEEP QUALITY: POOR / OK / GOOD / GREAT

STRESS LEVELS: NONE / LOW / MEDIUM / HIGH

HYDRATION: ☐ ☐ ☐ ☐ ☐ ☐ ☐ ☐

M / T / W / T / F / S / S   DATE:

Meal	Blood sugar levels		Notes
	TIME:		
FASTING			
	PRE	POST	
BREAKFAST	TIME:	TIME:	
LUNCH	TIME:	TIME:	
DINNER	TIME:	TIME:	
SNACKS			

WEIGHT:

EXERCISE:

SLEEP QUALITY: POOR / OK / GOOD / GREAT

STRESS LEVELS: NONE / LOW / MEDIUM / HIGH

HYDRATION: ☐ ☐ ☐ ☐ ☐ ☐ ☐

M / T / W / T / F / S / S   DATE:

Meal	Blood sugar levels		Notes
	TIME:		
FASTING			
	PRE	POST	
BREAKFAST	TIME:	TIME:	
LUNCH	TIME:	TIME:	
DINNER	TIME:	TIME:	
SNACKS			

WEIGHT:

EXERCISE:

SLEEP QUALITY: POOR / OK / GOOD / GREAT

STRESS LEVELS: NONE / LOW / MEDIUM / HIGH

HYDRATION: ▢ ▢ ▢ ▢ ▢ ▢ ▢ ▢

M / T / W / T / F / S / S   DATE:

Meal	Blood sugar levels		Notes
	TIME:		
FASTING	PRE	POST	
BREAKFAST	TIME:	TIME:	
LUNCH	TIME:	TIME:	
DINNER	TIME:	TIME:	
SNACKS			

WEIGHT:

EXERCISE:

SLEEP QUALITY: POOR / OK / GOOD / GREAT

STRESS LEVELS: NONE / LOW / MEDIUM / HIGH

HYDRATION: ☐ ☐ ☐ ☐ ☐ ☐ ☐ ☐

M / T / W / T / F / S / S   DATE:

Meal	Blood sugar levels		Notes
	TIME:		
FASTING			
BREAKFAST	PRE	POST	
	TIME:	TIME:	
LUNCH	TIME:	TIME:	
DINNER	TIME:	TIME:	
SNACKS	TIME:		

WEIGHT:

EXERCISE:

SLEEP QUALITY: POOR / OK / GOOD / GREAT

STRESS LEVELS: NONE / LOW / MEDIUM / HIGH

HYDRATION: ☐ ☐ ☐ ☐ ☐ ☐ ☐ ☐

M / T / W / T / F / S / S   DATE:

Meal	Blood sugar levels		Notes
FASTING	TIME:		
	PRE	POST	
BREAKFAST	TIME:	TIME:	
LUNCH	TIME:	TIME:	
DINNER	TIME:	TIME:	
SNACKS			
	WEIGHT:		
	EXERCISE:		

SLEEP QUALITY: POOR / OK / GOOD / GREAT

STRESS LEVELS: NONE / LOW / MEDIUM / HIGH

HYDRATION: ☐ ☐ ☐ ☐ ☐ ☐ ☐ ☐

M / T / W / T / F / S / S   DATE:

Meal	Blood sugar levels		Notes
	TIME:		
FASTING			
	PRE	POST	
BREAKFAST	TIME:	TIME:	
LUNCH	TIME:	TIME:	
DINNER	TIME:	TIME:	
SNACKS			
WEIGHT:			
EXERCISE:			

SLEEP QUALITY: POOR / OK / GOOD / GREAT

STRESS LEVELS: NONE / LOW / MEDIUM / HIGH

HYDRATION: ☐ ☐ ☐ ☐ ☐ ☐ ☐ ☐

M / T / W / T / F / S / S   DATE:

Meal	Blood sugar levels		Notes
	PRE	POST	
FASTING	TIME:		
BREAKFAST	TIME:	TIME:	
LUNCH	TIME:	TIME:	
DINNER	TIME:	TIME:	
SNACKS			

WEIGHT:

EXERCISE:

SLEEP QUALITY: POOR / OK / GOOD / GREAT

STRESS LEVELS: NONE / LOW / MEDIUM / HIGH

HYDRATION: ▢ ▢ ▢ ▢ ▢ ▢ ▢ ▢

M / T / W / T / F / S / S   DATE:

Meal	Blood sugar levels		Notes
FASTING	TIME:		
	PRE	POST	
BREAKFAST	TIME:	TIME:	
LUNCH	TIME:	TIME:	
DINNER	TIME:	TIME:	
SNACKS	TIME:		

WEIGHT:

EXERCISE:

SLEEP QUALITY: POOR / OK / GOOD / GREAT

STRESS LEVELS: NONE / LOW / MEDIUM / HIGH

HYDRATION: ▢ ▢ ▢ ▢ ▢ ▢ ▢ ▢

M / T / W / T / F / S / S   DATE:

Meal	Blood sugar levels		Notes
	TIME:		
FASTING			
	PRE	POST	
BREAKFAST	TIME:	TIME:	
LUNCH	TIME:	TIME:	
DINNER	TIME:	TIME:	
SNACKS	TIME:		

WEIGHT:

EXERCISE:

SLEEP QUALITY: POOR / OK / GOOD / GREAT

STRESS LEVELS: NONE / LOW / MEDIUM / HIGH

HYDRATION: ☐☐☐☐☐☐☐☐

M / T / W / T / F / S / S   DATE:

Meal	Blood sugar levels		Notes
	TIME:		
	PRE	POST	
FASTING			
BREAKFAST	TIME:	TIME:	
LUNCH	TIME:	TIME:	
DINNER	TIME:	TIME:	
SNACKS			

WEIGHT:

EXERCISE:

SLEEP QUALITY: POOR / OK / GOOD / GREAT

STRESS LEVELS: NONE / LOW / MEDIUM / HIGH

HYDRATION: ☐ ☐ ☐ ☐ ☐ ☐ ☐ ☐

M / T / W / T / F / S / S   DATE:

Meal	Blood sugar levels		Notes
FASTING	TIME:		
	PRE	POST	
BREAKFAST	TIME:	TIME:	
LUNCH	TIME:	TIME:	
DINNER	TIME:	TIME:	
SNACKS	TIME:		
	WEIGHT:		
SLEEP QUALITY: POOR / OK / GOOD / GREAT	EXERCISE:		
STRESS LEVELS: NONE / LOW / MEDIUM / HIGH			
HYDRATION: ▢▢▢▢▢▢▢▢			

M / T / W / T / F / S / S   DATE:

Meal	Blood sugar levels		Notes
FASTING	TIME:		
	PRE	POST	
BREAKFAST	TIME:	TIME:	
LUNCH	TIME:	TIME:	
DINNER	TIME:	TIME:	
SNACKS	TIME:		

WEIGHT:

EXERCISE:

SLEEP QUALITY: POOR / OK / GOOD / GREAT

STRESS LEVELS: NONE / LOW / MEDIUM / HIGH

HYDRATION: ☐ ☐ ☐ ☐ ☐ ☐ ☐ ☐

M / T / W / T / F / S / S   DATE:

Meal	Blood sugar levels		Notes
	TIME:		
FASTING			
	PRE	POST	
BREAKFAST	TIME:	TIME:	
LUNCH	TIME:	TIME:	
DINNER	TIME:	TIME:	
SNACKS			

WEIGHT:

EXERCISE:

SLEEP QUALITY: POOR / OK / GOOD / GREAT

STRESS LEVELS: NONE / LOW / MEDIUM / HIGH

HYDRATION: ☐ ☐ ☐ ☐ ☐ ☐ ☐ ☐

M / T / W / T / F / S / S   DATE:

Meal	Blood sugar levels		Notes
FASTING	TIME:		
	PRE	POST	
BREAKFAST	TIME:	TIME:	
LUNCH	TIME:	TIME:	
DINNER	TIME:	TIME:	
SNACKS			

WEIGHT:

EXERCISE:

SLEEP QUALITY: POOR / OK / GOOD / GREAT

STRESS LEVELS: NONE / LOW / MEDIUM / HIGH

HYDRATION: ▢ ▢ ▢ ▢ ▢ ▢ ▢

M / T / W / T / F / S / S   DATE:

Meal	Blood sugar levels		Notes
	PRE	POST	
FASTING	TIME:		
BREAKFAST	TIME:	TIME:	
LUNCH	TIME:	TIME:	
DINNER	TIME:	TIME:	
SNACKS	TIME:		

WEIGHT:

EXERCISE:

SLEEP QUALITY: POOR / OK / GOOD / GREAT

STRESS LEVELS: NONE / LOW / MEDIUM / HIGH

HYDRATION: ☐ ☐ ☐ ☐ ☐ ☐ ☐ ☐

M / T / W / T / F / S / S   DATE:

Meal	Blood sugar levels		Notes
	TIME:		
	PRE	POST	
FASTING			
BREAKFAST	TIME:	TIME:	
LUNCH	TIME:	TIME:	
DINNER	TIME:	TIME:	
SNACKS	TIME:		

WEIGHT:

EXERCISE:

SLEEP QUALITY: POOR / OK / GOOD / GREAT

STRESS LEVELS: NONE / LOW / MEDIUM / HIGH

HYDRATION: ▢ ▢ ▢ ▢ ▢ ▢ ▢ ▢

M / T / W / T / F / S / S   DATE:

Meal	Blood sugar levels			Notes
FASTING	TIME:			
BREAKFAST	PRE TIME:	POST TIME:		
LUNCH	TIME:	TIME:		
DINNER	TIME:	TIME:		
SNACKS	TIME:			

WEIGHT:

EXERCISE:

SLEEP QUALITY: POOR / OK / GOOD / GREAT

STRESS LEVELS: NONE / LOW / MEDIUM / HIGH

HYDRATION: ▢ ▢ ▢ ▢ ▢ ▢ ▢

M / T / W / T / F / S / S   DATE:

Meal	Blood sugar levels		Notes
	PRE	POST	
FASTING TIME:			
BREAKFAST	TIME:	TIME:	
LUNCH	TIME:	TIME:	
DINNER	TIME:	TIME:	
SNACKS			

WEIGHT:

EXERCISE:

SLEEP QUALITY: POOR / OK / GOOD / GREAT

STRESS LEVELS: NONE / LOW / MEDIUM / HIGH

HYDRATION: ▢ ▢ ▢ ▢ ▢ ▢ ▢ ▢

M / T / W / T / F / S / S   DATE:

Meal	Blood sugar levels		Notes
	PRE	POST	
FASTING	TIME:		
BREAKFAST	TIME:	TIME:	
LUNCH	TIME:	TIME:	
DINNER	TIME:	TIME:	
SNACKS			

WEIGHT:

EXERCISE:

SLEEP QUALITY: POOR / OK / GOOD / GREAT

STRESS LEVELS: NONE / LOW / MEDIUM / HIGH

HYDRATION: ☐ ☐ ☐ ☐ ☐ ☐ ☐ ☐

M / T / W / T / F / S / S   DATE:

Meal	Blood sugar levels		Notes
FASTING	TIME:		
	PRE	POST	
BREAKFAST	TIME:	TIME:	
LUNCH	TIME:	TIME:	
DINNER	TIME:	TIME:	
SNACKS	TIME:		

SLEEP QUALITY: POOR / OK / GOOD / GREAT   WEIGHT:

STRESS LEVELS: NONE / LOW / MEDIUM / HIGH   EXERCISE:

HYDRATION: ▢ ▢ ▢ ▢ ▢ ▢ ▢ ▢

M / T / W / T / F / S / S   DATE:

Meal	Blood sugar levels		Notes
	PRE	POST	
FASTING	TIME:		
BREAKFAST	TIME:	TIME:	
LUNCH	TIME:	TIME:	
DINNER	TIME:	TIME:	
SNACKS	TIME:		

WEIGHT:

EXERCISE:

SLEEP QUALITY: POOR / OK / GOOD / GREAT

STRESS LEVELS: NONE / LOW / MEDIUM / HIGH

HYDRATION: ☐ ☐ ☐ ☐ ☐ ☐ ☐ ☐

M / T / W / T / F / S / S   · DATE:

Meal	Blood sugar levels		Notes
	TIME:		
FASTING			
	PRE	POST	
BREAKFAST	TIME:	TIME:	
LUNCH	TIME:	TIME:	
DINNER	TIME:	TIME:	
SNACKS			

SLEEP QUALITY: POOR / OK / GOOD / GREAT

STRESS LEVELS: NONE / LOW / MEDIUM / HIGH

HYDRATION: ☐ ☐ ☐ ☐ ☐ ☐ ☐ ☐

WEIGHT:

EXERCISE:

M / T / W / T / F / S / S   DATE:

Meal	Blood sugar levels		Notes
	PRE	POST	
FASTING	TIME:		
BREAKFAST	TIME:	TIME:	
LUNCH	TIME:	TIME:	
DINNER	TIME:	TIME:	
SNACKS	TIME:		

WEIGHT:

EXERCISE:

SLEEP QUALITY: POOR / OK / GOOD / GREAT

STRESS LEVELS: NONE / LOW / MEDIUM / HIGH

HYDRATION: ☐ ☐ ☐ ☐ ☐ ☐ ☐ ☐

M / T / W / T / F / S / S   DATE:

Meal	Blood sugar levels		Notes
FASTING	TIME:		
	PRE	POST	
BREAKFAST	TIME:	TIME:	
LUNCH	TIME:	TIME:	
DINNER	TIME:	TIME:	
SNACKS	TIME:		

SLEEP QUALITY: POOR / OK / GOOD / GREAT   WEIGHT:

STRESS LEVELS: NONE / LOW / MEDIUM / HIGH   EXERCISE:

HYDRATION: ☐ ☐ ☐ ☐ ☐ ☐ ☐ ☐

M / T / W / T / F / S / S   DATE:

Meal	Blood sugar levels		Notes
	TIME:		
FASTING			
	PRE	POST	
	TIME:	TIME:	
BREAKFAST			
	TIME:	TIME:	
LUNCH			
	TIME:	TIME:	
DINNER			
	TIME:		
SNACKS			

WEIGHT:

EXERCISE:

SLEEP QUALITY: POOR / OK / GOOD / GREAT

STRESS LEVELS: NONE / LOW / MEDIUM / HIGH

HYDRATION: ☐ ☐ ☐ ☐ ☐ ☐ ☐

M / T / W / T / F / S / S   DATE:

Meal	Blood sugar levels		Notes
FASTING	TIME:		
	PRE	POST	
BREAKFAST	TIME:	TIME:	
LUNCH	TIME:	TIME:	
DINNER	TIME:	TIME:	
SNACKS			

WEIGHT:

EXERCISE:

SLEEP QUALITY: POOR / OK / GOOD / GREAT

STRESS LEVELS: NONE / LOW / MEDIUM / HIGH

HYDRATION: ☐ ☐ ☐ ☐ ☐ ☐ ☐ ☐

M / T / W / T / F / S / S   DATE:

Meal	Blood sugar levels		Notes
FASTING	TIME:		
BREAKFAST	PRE TIME:	POST TIME:	
LUNCH	TIME:	TIME:	
DINNER	TIME:	TIME:	
SNACKS	TIME:		

WEIGHT:

EXERCISE:

SLEEP QUALITY: POOR / OK / GOOD / GREAT

STRESS LEVELS: NONE / LOW / MEDIUM / HIGH

HYDRATION: ▢ ▢ ▢ ▢ ▢ ▢

M / T / W / T / F / S / S   DATE:

Meal	Blood sugar levels		Notes
FASTING	TIME:		
BREAKFAST	TIME: PRE	TIME: POST	
LUNCH	TIME:	TIME:	
DINNER	TIME:	TIME:	
SNACKS			

WEIGHT:

EXERCISE:

SLEEP QUALITY: POOR / OK / GOOD / GREAT

STRESS LEVELS: NONE / LOW / MEDIUM / HIGH

HYDRATION: ☐ ☐ ☐ ☐ ☐ ☐ ☐ ☐

M / T / W / T / F / S / S   DATE:

Meal	Blood sugar levels		Notes
	TIME:		
FASTING			
	PRE	POST	
BREAKFAST	TIME:	TIME:	
LUNCH	TIME:	TIME:	
DINNER	TIME:	TIME:	
SNACKS			
WEIGHT:			
EXERCISE:			

SLEEP QUALITY: POOR / OK / GOOD / GREAT

STRESS LEVELS: NONE / LOW / MEDIUM / HIGH

HYDRATION: ☐ ☐ ☐ ☐ ☐ ☐ ☐

M / T / W / T / F / S / S   DATE:

Meal	Blood sugar levels		Notes
	PRE	POST	
FASTING	TIME:		
BREAKFAST	TIME:	TIME:	
LUNCH	TIME:	TIME:	
DINNER	TIME:	TIME:	
SNACKS			

WEIGHT:

EXERCISE:

SLEEP QUALITY: POOR / OK / GOOD / GREAT

STRESS LEVELS: NONE / LOW / MEDIUM / HIGH

HYDRATION: ☐ ☐ ☐ ☐ ☐ ☐ ☐ ☐

M / T / W / T / F / S / S   DATE:

Meal	Blood sugar levels		Notes
FASTING	TIME:		
BREAKFAST	PRE	POST	
	TIME:	TIME:	
LUNCH			
	TIME:	TIME:	
DINNER			
	TIME:	TIME:	
SNACKS			

WEIGHT:

EXERCISE:

SLEEP QUALITY: POOR / OK / GOOD / GREAT

STRESS LEVELS: NONE / LOW / MEDIUM / HIGH

HYDRATION: ☐ ☐ ☐ ☐ ☐ ☐ ☐ ☐

M / T / W / T / F / S / S   DATE:

Meal	Blood sugar levels		Notes
FASTING	TIME:		
	PRE	POST	
BREAKFAST	TIME:	TIME:	
LUNCH	TIME:	TIME:	
DINNER	TIME:	TIME:	
SNACKS	TIME:		

WEIGHT:

EXERCISE:

SLEEP QUALITY: POOR / OK / GOOD / GREAT

STRESS LEVELS: NONE / LOW / MEDIUM / HIGH

HYDRATION: ☐ ☐ ☐ ☐ ☐ ☐ ☐ ☐

M / T / W / T / F / S / S   DATE:

Meal	Blood sugar levels		Notes
FASTING	TIME:		
BREAKFAST	PRE	POST	
	TIME:	TIME:	
LUNCH	TIME:	TIME:	
DINNER	TIME:	TIME:	
SNACKS			

WEIGHT:

EXERCISE:

SLEEP QUALITY: POOR / OK / GOOD / GREAT

STRESS LEVELS: NONE / LOW / MEDIUM / HIGH

HYDRATION: ▢ ▢ ▢ ▢ ▢ ▢ ▢ ▢

M / T / W / T / F / S / S   DATE:

Meal	Blood sugar levels			Notes
	TIME:			
FASTING				
		PRE	POST	
BREAKFAST	TIME:		TIME:	
LUNCH	TIME:		TIME:	
DINNER	TIME:		TIME:	
SNACKS	TIME:			

WEIGHT:

EXERCISE:

SLEEP QUALITY: POOR / OK / GOOD / GREAT

STRESS LEVELS: NONE / LOW / MEDIUM / HIGH

HYDRATION: ☐ ☐ ☐ ☐ ☐ ☐ ☐ ☐

M / T / W / T / F / S / S   DATE:

Meal	Blood sugar levels		Notes
FASTING	TIME:		
	PRE	POST	
BREAKFAST	TIME:	TIME:	
LUNCH	TIME:	TIME:	
DINNER	TIME:	TIME:	
SNACKS	TIME:		
WEIGHT:			
EXERCISE:			

SLEEP QUALITY: POOR / OK / GOOD / GREAT

STRESS LEVELS: NONE / LOW / MEDIUM / HIGH

HYDRATION: ▢ ▢ ▢ ▢ ▢ ▢ ▢

M / T / W / T / F / S / S   DATE:

Meal	Blood sugar levels		Notes
FASTING	TIME:		
BREAKFAST	PRE	POST	
	TIME:	TIME:	
LUNCH	TIME:	TIME:	
DINNER	TIME:	TIME:	
SNACKS			

WEIGHT:

EXERCISE:

SLEEP QUALITY: POOR / OK / GOOD / GREAT

STRESS LEVELS: NONE / LOW / MEDIUM / HIGH

HYDRATION: ☐ ☐ ☐ ☐ ☐ ☐ ☐ ☐

M / T / W / T / F / S / S   DATE:

Meal	Blood sugar levels		Notes
FASTING	TIME:		
BREAKFAST	PRE	POST	
	TIME:	TIME:	
LUNCH	TIME:	TIME:	
DINNER	TIME:	TIME:	
SNACKS	TIME:		

WEIGHT:

EXERCISE:

SLEEP QUALITY: POOR / OK / GOOD / GREAT

STRESS LEVELS: NONE / LOW / MEDIUM / HIGH

HYDRATION: ▢ ▢ ▢ ▢ ▢ ▢ ▢ ▢

M / T / W / T / F / S / S   DATE:

Meal	Blood sugar levels		Notes
	PRE	POST	
FASTING	TIME:		
BREAKFAST	TIME:	TIME:	
LUNCH	TIME:	TIME:	
DINNER	TIME:	TIME:	
SNACKS	TIME:		

SLEEP QUALITY: POOR / OK / GOOD / GREAT

STRESS LEVELS: NONE / LOW / MEDIUM / HIGH

HYDRATION: ▢ ▢ ▢ ▢ ▢ ▢ ▢ ▢

WEIGHT:

EXERCISE:

M / T / W / T / F / S / S   DATE:

Meal	Blood sugar levels		Notes
	PRE	POST	
FASTING	TIME:		
BREAKFAST	TIME:	TIME:	
LUNCH	TIME:	TIME:	
DINNER	TIME:	TIME:	
SNACKS			

WEIGHT:

EXERCISE:

SLEEP QUALITY: POOR / OK / GOOD / GREAT

STRESS LEVELS: NONE / LOW / MEDIUM / HIGH

HYDRATION: ☐ ☐ ☐ ☐ ☐ ☐ ☐ ☐

M / T / W / T / F / S / S   DATE:

Meal	Blood sugar levels		Notes
FASTING	TIME:		
	PRE	POST	
BREAKFAST	TIME:	TIME:	
LUNCH	TIME:	TIME:	
DINNER	TIME:	TIME:	
SNACKS	TIME:		

WEIGHT:

EXERCISE:

SLEEP QUALITY: POOR / OK / GOOD / GREAT

STRESS LEVELS: NONE / LOW / MEDIUM / HIGH

HYDRATION: ▢ ▢ ▢ ▢ ▢ ▢ ▢ ▢

M / T / W / T / F / S / S   DATE:

Meal	Blood sugar levels		Notes
FASTING	TIME:		
BREAKFAST	PRE	POST	
	TIME:	TIME:	
LUNCH	TIME:	TIME:	
DINNER	TIME:	TIME:	
SNACKS			

WEIGHT:

EXERCISE:

SLEEP QUALITY: POOR / OK / GOOD / GREAT

STRESS LEVELS: NONE / LOW / MEDIUM / HIGH

HYDRATION: ▢ ▢ ▢ ▢ ▢ ▢ ▢ ▢

M / T / W / T / F / S / S   DATE:

Meal	Blood sugar levels		Notes
		PRE	POST	
FASTING	TIME:		
BREAKFAST	TIME:	TIME:	
LUNCH	TIME:		
DINNER	TIME:	TIME:	
SNACKS			

WEIGHT:

EXERCISE:

SLEEP QUALITY: POOR / OK / GOOD / GREAT

STRESS LEVELS: NONE / LOW / MEDIUM / HIGH

HYDRATION: ⬡ ⬡ ⬡ ⬡ ⬡ ⬡ ⬡ ⬡

M / T / W / T / F / S / S   DATE:

Meal	Blood sugar levels		Notes
	PRE	POST	
FASTING	TIME:		
BREAKFAST	TIME:	TIME:	
LUNCH	TIME:	TIME:	
DINNER	TIME:	TIME:	
SNACKS			

SLEEP QUALITY: POOR / OK / GOOD / GREAT

STRESS LEVELS: NONE / LOW / MEDIUM / HIGH

HYDRATION: ☐ ☐ ☐ ☐ ☐ ☐ ☐ ☐

WEIGHT:

EXERCISE:

M / T / W / T / F / S / S   DATE:

Meal	Blood sugar levels		Notes
	TIME:		
FASTING	PRE	POST	
BREAKFAST	TIME:	TIME:	
LUNCH	TIME:	TIME:	
DINNER	TIME:	TIME:	
SNACKS			

WEIGHT:

EXERCISE:

SLEEP QUALITY: POOR / OK / GOOD / GREAT

STRESS LEVELS: NONE / LOW / MEDIUM / HIGH

HYDRATION: ▢ ▢ ▢ ▢ ▢ ▢ ▢ ▢

M / T / W / T / F / S / S   DATE:

Meal	Blood sugar levels		Notes
	TIME:		
	PRE	POST	
FASTING			
BREAKFAST	TIME:	TIME:	
LUNCH	TIME:	TIME:	
DINNER	TIME:	TIME:	
SNACKS			

WEIGHT:

EXERCISE:

SLEEP QUALITY: POOR / OK / GOOD / GREAT

STRESS LEVELS: NONE / LOW / MEDIUM / HIGH

HYDRATION: ☐ ☐ ☐ ☐ ☐ ☐ ☐ ☐

M / T / W / T / F / S / S   DATE:

Meal	Blood sugar levels		Notes
FASTING	TIME:		
	PRE	POST	
BREAKFAST	TIME:	TIME:	
LUNCH	TIME:	TIME:	
DINNER	TIME:	TIME:	
SNACKS	TIME:		

WEIGHT:

EXERCISE:

SLEEP QUALITY: POOR / OK / GOOD / GREAT

STRESS LEVELS: NONE / LOW / MEDIUM / HIGH

HYDRATION: ▢ ▢ ▢ ▢ ▢ ▢ ▢ ▢

M / T / W / T / F / S / S   DATE:

Meal	Blood sugar levels		Notes
	PRE	POST	
FASTING	TIME:		
BREAKFAST	TIME:	TIME:	
LUNCH	TIME:	TIME:	
DINNER	TIME:	TIME:	
SNACKS			

WEIGHT:

EXERCISE:

SLEEP QUALITY: POOR / OK / GOOD / GREAT

STRESS LEVELS: NONE / LOW / MEDIUM / HIGH

HYDRATION: ☐ ☐ ☐ ☐ ☐ ☐ ☐ ☐

M / T / W / T / F / S / S   DATE:

Meal	Blood sugar levels		Notes
	TIME:		
FASTING			
	PRE	POST	
BREAKFAST			
	TIME:	TIME:	
LUNCH	TIME:	TIME:	
DINNER	TIME:	TIME:	
SNACKS			

WEIGHT:

EXERCISE:

SLEEP QUALITY: POOR / OK / GOOD / GREAT

STRESS LEVELS: NONE / LOW / MEDIUM / HIGH

HYDRATION: ☐ ☐ ☐ ☐ ☐ ☐ ☐ ☐

M / T / W / T / F / S / S   DATE:

Meal	Blood sugar levels		Notes
	PRE	POST	
FASTING	TIME:		
BREAKFAST	TIME:	TIME:	
LUNCH	TIME:	TIME:	
DINNER	TIME:	TIME:	
SNACKS			

WEIGHT:

EXERCISE:

SLEEP QUALITY: POOR / OK / GOOD / GREAT

STRESS LEVELS: NONE / LOW / MEDIUM / HIGH

HYDRATION: ☐ ☐ ☐ ☐ ☐ ☐ ☐ ☐

M / T / W / T / F / S / S   DATE:

Meal	Blood sugar levels		Notes
	TIME:		
	PRE	POST	
FASTING			
BREAKFAST	TIME:	TIME:	
LUNCH	TIME:	TIME:	
DINNER	TIME:	TIME:	
SNACKS	TIME:		

SLEEP QUALITY: POOR / OK / GOOD / GREAT   WEIGHT:

STRESS LEVELS: NONE / LOW / MEDIUM / HIGH   EXERCISE:

HYDRATION: ☐ ☐ ☐ ☐ ☐ ☐ ☐

M / T / W / T / F / S / S   DATE:

Meal	Blood sugar levels			Notes
FASTING	TIME:			
BREAKFAST		PRE TIME:	POST TIME:	
LUNCH	TIME:		TIME:	
DINNER	TIME:		TIME:	
SNACKS	TIME:			

WEIGHT:

EXERCISE:

SLEEP QUALITY: POOR / OK / GOOD / GREAT

STRESS LEVELS: NONE / LOW / MEDIUM / HIGH

HYDRATION: ☐ ☐ ☐ ☐ ☐ ☐ ☐

M / T / W / T / F / S / S   DATE:

Meal	Blood sugar levels		Notes
	TIME:		
FASTING			
	PRE	POST	
BREAKFAST	TIME:	TIME:	
LUNCH	TIME:	TIME:	
DINNER	TIME:	TIME:	
SNACKS			

WEIGHT:

EXERCISE:

SLEEP QUALITY: POOR / OK / GOOD / GREAT

STRESS LEVELS: NONE / LOW / MEDIUM / HIGH

HYDRATION: ▢ ▢ ▢ ▢ ▢ ▢ ▢ ▢

M / T / W / T / F / S / S   DATE:

Meal	Blood sugar levels		Notes
	TIME:		
	PRE	POST	
FASTING			
BREAKFAST	TIME:	TIME:	
LUNCH	TIME:	TIME:	
DINNER	TIME:	TIME:	
SNACKS			

WEIGHT:

EXERCISE:

SLEEP QUALITY: POOR / OK / GOOD / GREAT

STRESS LEVELS: NONE / LOW / MEDIUM / HIGH

HYDRATION: ▢ ▢ ▢ ▢ ▢ ▢ ▢ ▢

M / T / W / T / F / S / S   DATE:

Meal	Blood sugar levels		Notes
FASTING	TIME:		
	PRE	POST	
BREAKFAST	TIME:	TIME:	
LUNCH	TIME:	TIME:	
DINNER	TIME:	TIME:	
SNACKS			

WEIGHT:

EXERCISE:

SLEEP QUALITY: POOR / OK / GOOD / GREAT

STRESS LEVELS: NONE / LOW / MEDIUM / HIGH

HYDRATION: ▢ ▢ ▢ ▢ ▢ ▢ ▢

M / T / W / T / F / S / S   DATE:

Meal	Blood sugar levels		Notes
	TIME:		
FASTING			
	PRE	POST	
BREAKFAST	TIME:	TIME:	
LUNCH	TIME:	TIME:	
DINNER	TIME:	TIME:	
SNACKS			

WEIGHT:

EXERCISE:

SLEEP QUALITY: POOR / OK / GOOD / GREAT

STRESS LEVELS: NONE / LOW / MEDIUM / HIGH

HYDRATION: ▢ ▢ ▢ ▢ ▢ ▢ ▢ ▢

M / T / W / T / F / S / S   DATE:

Meal	Blood sugar levels		Notes
	TIME:		
	PRE	POST	
FASTING			
BREAKFAST	TIME:	TIME:	
LUNCH	TIME:	TIME:	
DINNER	TIME:	TIME:	
SNACKS	TIME:		

SLEEP QUALITY: POOR / OK / GOOD / GREAT   WEIGHT:

STRESS LEVELS: NONE / LOW / MEDIUM / HIGH   EXERCISE:

HYDRATION: ☐ ☐ ☐ ☐ ☐ ☐ ☐

M / T / W / T / F / S / S   DATE:

Meal	Blood sugar levels		Notes
		PRE	POST	
FASTING	TIME:		
BREAKFAST		TIME:	TIME:	
LUNCH		TIME:	TIME:	
DINNER		TIME:	TIME:	
SNACKS		TIME:		

SLEEP QUALITY: POOR / OK / GOOD / GREAT

STRESS LEVELS: NONE / LOW / MEDIUM / HIGH

HYDRATION: ▢ ▢ ▢ ▢ ▢ ▢ ▢ ▢

WEIGHT:

EXERCISE:

M / T / W / T / F / S / S   DATE:

Meal	Blood sugar levels		Notes
	TIME:		
	PRE	POST	
FASTING			
BREAKFAST	TIME:	TIME:	
LUNCH	TIME:	TIME:	
DINNER	TIME:	TIME:	
SNACKS			

WEIGHT:

EXERCISE:

SLEEP QUALITY: POOR / OK / GOOD / GREAT

STRESS LEVELS: NONE / LOW / MEDIUM / HIGH

HYDRATION: ▢ ▢ ▢ ▢ ▢ ▢ ▢ ▢

M / T / W / T / F / S / S   DATE:

Meal	Blood sugar levels		Notes
	TIME:		
FASTING			
	PRE	POST	
BREAKFAST	TIME:	TIME:	
LUNCH	TIME:	TIME:	
DINNER	TIME:	TIME:	
SNACKS			

WEIGHT:

EXERCISE:

SLEEP QUALITY: POOR / OK / GOOD / GREAT

STRESS LEVELS: NONE / LOW / MEDIUM / HIGH

HYDRATION: ▢ ▢ ▢ ▢ ▢ ▢ ▢ ▢

M / T / W / T / F / S / S   DATE:

Meal	Blood sugar levels		Notes
	TIME:		
	PRE	POST	
FASTING			
BREAKFAST	TIME:	TIME:	
LUNCH	TIME:	TIME:	
DINNER	TIME:	TIME:	
SNACKS			

WEIGHT:

EXERCISE:

SLEEP QUALITY: POOR / OK / GOOD / GREAT

STRESS LEVELS: NONE / LOW / MEDIUM / HIGH

HYDRATION: ☐ ☐ ☐ ☐ ☐ ☐ ☐ ☐

M / T / W / T / F / S / S   DATE:

Meal	Blood sugar levels		Notes
	TIME:		
	PRE	POST	
FASTING			
BREAKFAST	TIME:	TIME:	
LUNCH	TIME:	TIME:	
DINNER	TIME:	TIME:	
SNACKS			

WEIGHT:

EXERCISE:

SLEEP QUALITY: POOR / OK / GOOD / GREAT

STRESS LEVELS: NONE / LOW / MEDIUM / HIGH

HYDRATION: ☐ ☐ ☐ ☐ ☐ ☐ ☐ ☐

M / T / W / T / F / S / S   DATE:

Meal	Blood sugar levels		Notes
FASTING	TIME:		
BREAKFAST	PRE	POST	
	TIME:	TIME:	
LUNCH	TIME:	TIME:	
DINNER	TIME:	TIME:	
SNACKS			

WEIGHT:

EXERCISE:

SLEEP QUALITY: POOR / OK / GOOD / GREAT

STRESS LEVELS: NONE / LOW / MEDIUM / HIGH

HYDRATION: ▯ ▯ ▯ ▯ ▯ ▯ ▯ ▯

M / T / W / T / F / S / S   DATE:

Meal	Blood sugar levels		Notes
	TIME:		
FASTING			
	PRE	POST	
BREAKFAST	TIME:	TIME:	
LUNCH	TIME:	TIME:	
DINNER	TIME:	TIME:	
SNACKS			

WEIGHT:

EXERCISE:

SLEEP QUALITY: POOR / OK / GOOD / GREAT

STRESS LEVELS: NONE / LOW / MEDIUM / HIGH

HYDRATION: ☐ ☐ ☐ ☐ ☐ ☐ ☐ ☐

Made in United States
North Haven, CT
11 December 2024

62207006R00095